Fitness Planner

Author: Stefan Bercea

This fitness planner has been created to offer support and guidance for beginners, people wanting to return to training in the gym and people recovering from an accident.

The planner focuses specifically on the motivation/ reason for which an individual should train and defines it as a goal to be achieved. The planner progresses into offering information and recommendations on how training should be approached, depending on chosen goal, by giving example and beginners training routines. The planner further progresses into discussing the idea of "dieting" and prompts readers towards a healthy challenge encouraging them to adopt a lifestyle and abandon the idea of dieting. The planner concludes by prompting readers to create a visual representation of their goal, training and eating lifestyle as a motivational tool for their fitness journey.

Page intentionally left blank

Your Fitness Companion

Find your motivation

- Build Muscle, Be Athletic or Become Powerful (M.A.P.)

How to train

- Find a training split
- Right amount of sets
- Right amount of reps
- Find the best exercises
- Big groups
- Arms
- Also, important
- Don't forget about abs

What to eat

- Test yourself by elimination

- Sugar, Milk, Gluten, Processed foods

- Stay away from diets

You design your plan

- Goal + Training + Food

Find your motivation

In regards with your fitness/ health journey it does not matter where you are in life, it matters what you want to achieve. There are three primary targets on which you can focus to improve and achieve your goals. Those are building Muscle, being Athletic or becoming more Powerful, we are going to call this M.A.P. By choosing one over the other does not imply that one is superior to the other two. By choosing one goal, will enable you to achieve that goal faster rather than focusing on all three of them at the same time or two goals at the same time.

Your goal will be and should be different than anyone else, therefore firstly **do not compare yourself** with anyone, not even yourself.

Here is a quick way to decide how to choose what is more important for you:

Step one – Put the best clothes that you have on and have a look in the mirror. After this, ask yourself if you would like to look bigger, and if seeing yourself a bit bigger in the mirror will make you a bit happier. If the answer is YES, hold on to that answer at the moment and go to Step two. If the answer is NO, it means that you don't need to build more muscle. Go to Step two see if that should be your goal.

Step two – Go on the floor and perform a push up, immediately after, perform a squat. Take a minute to think how that made you feel and ask yourself if you would feel better and happier by becoming stronger/ more powerful. If the answer is NO than gaining more strength is not your goal. If your answer is YES, gaining strength might be your goal. Take in consideration your answers at the previous step, we have four scenarios:

A) – Answering NO to both questions.

B) – Answering NO to the first step and YES to the second one.

C) – Answering YES to the first step and NO to the second one.

D) – Answering YES to both questions.

A) You are mostly looking be either more athletic or maintain the way that you look. You can skip Step three and decide between maintain the way that you look or becoming more athletic.

B) At the moment your goal might be either becoming more powerful or becoming more athletic. You should definitely, go to step three to decide your goal.

C) At the moment, your goal might be either building more muscle or becoming more athletic. You should definitely, go to step three to decide your goal.

D) If you answered Yes to both questions, you now have the hard decision to choose which one is more important for you. Therefore, what is more important to you building muscle or being stronger? Once you decided, go to step three.

Step three – If you are here, it means that you are still deciding between either building muscle or becoming more powerful and becoming more athletic. At this stage you should look in the mirror without your shirt on and then ask yourself if by losing some weight you would feel happier. If the answer is NO, then becoming more athletic is not your goal. You should focus on the goal which decided at the previous step (either building muscle or becoming more powerful). If your answer is YES, you need to decide which goal is more important to you, think about which one will make you feel happier.

Regardless of your GOAL this planner will support you in achieving it. The next section focuses on how to train in the gym, it covers how to choose a training split for yourself, the appropriate number of repetitions and sets for your goal, best exercises and gives you a short introduction on muscle biomechanics.

How to Train

1. Training split:

When you train intensively to achieve your goal it is important to consider a **training split**. A training split is mostly defined by the amount of day which you can allocate to train in a week. It is quite common to hear arguments that one training split is better than another. In reality, everyone is different, we have different careers, jobs and we manage our time quite differently. Theoretically a person could train from one day per week to training every single day. Training intensively for every single day in week might not be optimum for recovery and may potentially lead to injuries in the long run. If you consider training for seven days a week, please be mindful of your recovery, injuries, and social life. Therefore, in this section we are going to go through splits covering one day week up to six days a week.

One day split.

Training one day per week can be beneficial for some people. If you have not been to the gym in a long time or if you are coming back to the gym after a long hiatus from an injury. Coming back for just one day could be exactly what you need. Having one day to work out can feel a bit tricky. My recommendations:

- If you are trying to build muscle and you are at the beginning or coming back from an injury, take this opportunity to build your mind muscle connection. Try to focus on five maybe six movements which target big muscle groups (chest, back, legs) and start building your foundation.

- If you are trying to lose some weight and become more athletic, this can be your opportunity to start with some cardio. If you haven't done anything in the past month and you looking at a way to start, think about this. If you do this one day a week of cardio for, let's say one month, you will achieve four cardio sessions.
- If your goal is to gain some strength and you only have one day free you can still do something. I would recommend you take this day to get comfortable with the movements and build your confidence.

Two-day split.

Two days is better than one, and possibly this is something that you can progress from one day a week, or you go straight into it. Regardless having an extra day to go and train gives you more benefits than training only once a week. My recommendations:

- If you are trying to build muscle, having two days a week this gives you the chances two train a bit differently. You can potentially split those days in an Upper/Lower body split (Chest, Back, Arms / Legs, Calves, Abs) or have two days in which you do a bit of everything (Full body split)
- If you are trying to lose some weight, I would recommend that you use one of the days for cardio and the other day for weight training. This way you can get the benefits of both in your training.

- If you are trying to build some strength, I recommend you take in account your form. Strength comes on equal ability with being able to perform the moves in a safe way. Therefore, I recommend allocating both days on basic movements and give yourself time to rest between the days, consider two to three days in between training days.

Three-day splits

Before we move on to three-day splits, it important to acknowledge that training once or twice a week is not the most beneficial way to train for any of your goals. Unless you are coming from an injury, are in a recovery period or you are extremely busy you should aim to train at least three or more times a week. Training three times a week gives you the flexibility and the minimum time to focus on your goal. My recommendations:

- If you are training to build muscle you should consider either a Full body split, as discussed in the above paragraphs you can target a bit of everything or you can choose a Push Pull Legs split. A Push Pull Legs split focuses on a different element of training in each day and it allows you to focus.
- If you are looking to lose weight mixing cardio and weights would be the most beneficial and effective to approach your goal. I would recommend a two-day training with weights, consider an Upper/ Lower split, and a day of cardio.
- If you are looking to build strength choosing a Full Body routine will help you improve your overall strength. A good way to schedule this would be by training every

other day and giving yourself a free weekend.

Four-day splits

Considering you have four days to train you can work towards achieving your goal quite strategically. Consider your days off, and how you can use that recovery in your advantage. You have three days off, do you need all three of them one after the other, or maybe you can arrange them differently. My recommendations:

- If you are training for muscle, you should consider four days of Full body training followed by three days of rest or maybe and Upper/Lower split. One whey to consider and Upper/ Lower split would be Upper day, Lower day, Rest Day, Upper day, Lower day, Rest Day, Rest Day.

- If you are training to lose weight, I recommend you mix weight training with cardio. In this case combining a Push, Pull, Legs split with one day of cardio can help you achieve your goal. Consider having a rest day after three days of training, follow this with your cardio day and then give yourself two days to recover.

- If you are training for strength and have four days when you can train, my recommendation is to focus on each big group once (Chest, Back and Legs) and use the fourth day to work on complimentary exercises to improve strength and stability. Here is an example: Leg Day, Back day, Rest, Rest, Chest Day, Complimentary day, Rest Day. In your complimentary day you should work towards improving other muscle groups that support you in your main lifts (calves, abs, shoulders, etc). Try to prioritise the groups which need this the most.

Five-day splits

Moving forward into more time demanding and rewarding routines, it's important to acknowledge that three to four days routine are great for beginners and intermediate level of training. Allocating five or six day a week to training with intensity will get you closer to your than three or four days, but you need to consider your recovery. If you are not recovering well enough from training with five- or six-day splits, you should consider changing your training to something that optimises your recovery. Now I consider five- and six-day split to be for advanced and intermediate level. My recommendations:

- If you are trying to build muscle your recovery is extremely important and with two days to rest, it is important that you use those to your advantage. One example of this would be using an Upper/Lower routine for four days followed by a rest day, followed by an either an Upper or Lower day (depending on what groups you need to prioritise) and then followed by a rest day. Example: Upper Day, Lower Day, Upper Day, Lower Day, Rest Day, Upper Day, Rest Day. Another style of training is by taking the rest days together for example if you are using a Push Pull Legs routine you can keep the two days together. Here is an example of this: Push Day, Pull Day, Leg Day, Push Day, Pull Day, Rest Day, Rest Day. Now the extra Push and Pull days are added to better stimulate those muscle groups.

Remember everyone is different, therefore you might choose that you need a Leg Day and a Push Day. Take in consideration your recovery, if you have a group which needs a longer period to recover it is okay to train that once a week, and if you have groups which recover quick enough you can train them twice a week.

- If you are training to lose weight my recommendation is to alternate between training days and cardio days. A heavy cardio routine would have three cardio days and two training days, for which I would recommend a Full body routine, the reverse can be as effective if you train with high intensity, having three full body days and two cardio days. Those would look like this: Cardio Day, Full Body Day, Cardio Day, Full Body Day, Cardio Day, Rest Day, Rest Day or

Full Body Day, Cardio Day, Full Body Day, Cardio Days, Full Body Day Rest Day, Rest Day.

- If you are trying to build some strength you need to optimise your recovery, this might mean for you giving yourself the time to recover from heavy lift. This is where the idea of a Bro split would be actually beneficial. By training at a very high intensity and allowing your body to recover you can achieve your goal. Consider training the big groups first Chest, Back, Legs and then use the other two days to strengthen your main lifts with an Arm Day and Core Day. Your Chest, Back, Leg Days should focus on compound movements which allow you to build more strength such as pressing, pulling, pushing, etc. and bring in your complimentary days should focus on movements which will improve your main lift. Therefore, think which movements will support with squatting, pushing, or pulling more weight and use those as the basis of you Core Day and Arm Day.

Six-day splits

When you train with high intensity for six days in a week it can become problematic in terms of recovery. Therefore, to get the most benefits out of your training availability it is important to listen to your body and make sure you recover well. My recommendations:

- If you are trying to build muscle, follow a routine which allows you to hit each group twice a week. For example, a Push Pull Legs routine would allow you to target each group twice a week and you can make slight alteration to each session to focus on what you want to obtain. This would look like this: Push Day, Pull Day, Leg Day, Push Day, Pull Day, Leg Day, Rest Day. On the second time training the same group focus on movements which compliment your first training.

- If you are training to lose some weight a six-day split gives you the opportunity to pair equal number of cardio days with training days, for which I recommend Push, Pull, Legs routine, or keep two cardio days and use the other four days for training with weights, for which I recommend an Upper/Lower routine. Those would look like this Push Day, Cardio

Day, Pull Day, Cardio Day, Legs Day, Cardio Day, Rest Day or Upper Day, Lower Day, Cardio Day, Upper Day, Lower Day, Cardio Day, Rest Day.

- For strength building you should focus on the functionality of the muscles. An example of this is considering your Chest it has primarily two movements with are pushing and bringing the arms across (imagine a cable fly). You can split your Chest Day in two, one focusing on pushing and the other one on flyes. Similarly, you can do the same with your Back and Legs, by splitting them into the movements which you are focusing to get stronger. This routine would look like this Chest

Day, Back Day, Legs Day, Chest Day,
Back Day, Legs Day, Rest Day.

What is the right amount of Sets and Repetitions?

Considering an exercise such as a Chest press or Cable fly, by executing the movement once you are performing one repetition. Most commonly within training out people choose to use between five and twelve repetitions. After performing a number of repetitions, let's say ten, people will stop, marking their first set of ten repetitions and then continue to perform usually somewhere between three to five sets of ten repetitions each. There are various techniques which can make sets more effective, such as drop sets and super sets. Which we will discuss later. The graph bellow illustrates the amount of volume which results by combining the most common

number of sets and number of repetitions.

Sets	3	4	5
Reps			
1	3	4	5
3	9	12	15
5	15	20	25
8	24	32	40
10	30	40	50
12	36	48	60
15	45	60	75
20	60	80	100
25	75	100	125

○
Strength sets/reps by Total output

○
Building muscle sets/reps by Total output

●
Athletic sets/reps by Total output

Sets of one repetition are considered a PR (personal record) and together with sets of three and five repetitions are considerate to be dedicated for building strength. The expectation when performing sets of one, three and five is that you will use high weights which will only allow you to perform a small number of repetitions. Sets of eight to twelve repetitions are often associated with building muscle as they allow you to lift high enough weights more frequently. This leaves sets of fifteen, twenty and twenty-five to be associated with more athletic movements, for example skipping, doing laps, boxing. My consideration within choosing the right amount of sets and repetitions comes from the total output. In other words, what do I get by performing this amount of sets and repetitions. The above table represents the consideration of this e-book when referring to types of sets either as athletic, building muscle or strength. Depending on your own goal which you decided earlier you can use this table to decide the amount of sets and repetitions for your training. My recommendation for beginners is:

- For strength development 3 Stets of 10 repetitions (3X10)
- For muscle building 4 Sets of 8 repetitions (4X8)
- For losing weight 5 Sets of 15 repetitions (5X15)

Regardless of your goal it is important to consider the weight in relationship with the number of repetitions you are performing. Consider any exercise, for example the chest press, and three set routines presented above. In the case of strength development sets you will want to perform with a weight which allows you to do only ten repetitions. You feel have chosen a weight which allows you to perform more than ten you should increase the weight. This applies to muscle building and athletic sets.

What should you train and what exercises should you perform?

Big Groups

As a beginner you should focus on those three groups: Chest, Back and Legs. This will help you develop the most aesthetic look of your body, build the most amount of strength and burn the most amount of calories. You should also move away from the idea of "best exercise for chest/back/legs" and focus on which movements you need to perform to target that specific muscle group.

The Chest muscle can be targeted by performing two movements. A pushing movement and a chest fly. You can perform the same movement in various forms for example, push-up, incline dumbbell press, decline barbell press, cable press, machine press, etc. All of them are pushing variation, and at the beginning of your fitness journey you should not get stuck into the mentality that one is better than the other. Consider those to be tools, and use what tools are available in your gym to your benefit. Also overusing the same tool does not guarantee you will get closer to your goal. Neither does over diversifying the tools that you use. If at the moment you find creating your own workout difficult, I want you to not worry. There is a section with detail training routines just before the "What should you eat?" section.

The Back muscles can be targeted through several movements such as pulling from above your head (imagine a pull-up or chin up), pulling in front of the body (example: seated cable rows, barbell row), straightening your back (deadlifts), and bringing your arms from above your head next to your body (pullover, cable pull overs). As a beginner I would recommend you focus on one or two of those movements depending on your goal and incorporate occasionally the other movements. If your goal is to build muscle recommend you focus on pull-ups and rows. For building strength deadlifts and rows should be your main focus. While trying to lose weight you should focus on deadlifts and pull-ups.

The Legs muscle can be targeted though flexion (imagine seated leg curls), deadlifts (example Romanian Deadlift), extension (seated leg extension) and pushing (squats). If your aim is building strength you should focus on squats and deadlifts, as they will bring you the most benefit. Those apply to losing weight as well, as both the squatting motion and deadlifting are compound movements (involve more muscle groups) would help you burn the most amount of calories. In regard to muscle building leg extension and curls can help you build more muscle.

Arms

When referring to arms within training with weight, it is often perceived that we refer to Shoulders, Triceps and Biceps. As you progress through your fitness journey you should incorporate dedicated exercises which target the development of those muscles. I would recommend focusing on those three groups possibly somewhere after two to three months of going to the gym or after at least twenty sessions in the gym.

Biceps can be targeted though the flexion of the arm within a range of position. The most extended position of the bicep is above your head and the most contracted position is behind your back. Starting from the most extended position the following exercises aim to show you the wide range in which you can train you biceps: Chin ups, Lateral high cable curls, Preacher curls, Inward hammer grip dumbbell curls, Dumbbell curls, Incline dumbbell curls. Regardless of your goal as a beginner you should focus on regular curls, those present the most benefits in terms of developing a good mind-muscle connection (feeling the muscle activating with each repetition).

Triceps can be targeted thought the extension of the arm within a range of positions. The most contracted position of the triceps is behind your back and the most elongated position is above your head. Starting from the most extended position the following exercises aim to show you the wide range in which you can train your triceps: Seated dumbbell triceps extension, Skull-crushers, Close grip EZ bar press, Rope pushdown, Parallel bar dips, Triceps kickbacks. My recommendation for beginners regardless of their aim is to focus on either an exercise such as the Close grip EZ bar press or Rope pushdown to establish a good mind muscle connection.

Shoulder can be targeted by focusing on their three ends (anterior head, lateral head, and posterior head). You can think of them as the one in front, lateral and at the back. Starting from the anterior to the posterior head the following exercises aim to show you the range in which you can train you shoulders: Dumbbell shoulder press, Shoulders lateral raises, and Dumbbell reverse fly. It is important to mention that all three heads of the shoulder are important. But if you were to pick one to start your fitness journey, I would recommend you start with the lateral head until you develop a god muscle connection.

Groups that are also important, but a lot of people forget about them

Don't forget about your Claves, Forearms and Trapezius muscle. In my opinion those are the most under-rated groups and should probably be given more importance, especially by intermediate lifters. As a beginner you should start to incorporate dedicated exercises to those groups possibly after your 40th session or depending on how often you train after five to six months. You should still take those groups in consideration prior to incorporating dedicated exercise and possibly choose compound movements that incorporate those groups in your training (squats, deadlifts, bench press).

Here are three exercises which you should incorporate for those groups, regardless of your goal. For traps you should perform Shrugs, for forearms you can perform Reverse wrist curls and for calves you can perform Seated Calf Raises. As you progress you should start to approach those muscle groups from different angles and different exercises.

Don't forget about your abdomen

Your abdomen is a muscle just like all the muscles discussed above and you should consider training it in a similar way you with train your chest and arms. The abdomen has several insertions which allow the muscle to contract. The following exercises aim to show you the wide range in which you can train your abdomen: Crunches, Dumbbell side bend, Reverse crunches, and Planks.

While you progress through your fitness journey you will learn that you should keep your abdomen engaged at all times to maximise the strength and control you have over the moves you perform. This means that to a certain degree you are "training" your abdomen on every single movement. With this being said you should start incorporating dedicated exercises for your abdomen from your 60th session or depending on how often you go to the gym might be your eight or nineth month.

Training Routines

Full Body

This routine is focused around the three big groups, and you can adapt it to your goal by choosing your own sets and repetitions.

Exercise 1: Machine Chest Press

Exercise 2: Machine Chest Fly

Exercise 3: Cable Lat Pulldown

Exercise 4: Seated Row Machine

Exercise 5: Leg Press Machine

Upper/ Lower

This routine focuses on the big groups while incorporating dedicated exercises for arms.

Upper Day

Exercise 1: Incline Dumbbell Chest Press

Exercise 2: Cable Lat Pulldown

Exercise 3: Dumbbell Lateral Raises for Shoulders

Exercise 4: Rope Pushdown

Exercise 5: Dumbbell Bicep Curls

Lower Day

Exercise 1: Machine Seated Leg Curls

Exercise 2: Dumbbell Romanian Deadlifts

Exercise 3: Machine Seated Leg Extension

Exercise 4: Dumbbell Goblet Squats

Exercise 5: Leg Press Machine

Push/ Pull/ Legs

This routine focuses on the big groups, arms, and includes dedicated exercises to traps, calves, and forearms.

Push

Exercise 1: Machine Chest Press

Exercise 2: Incline Dumbbell Chest Fly

Exercise 3: Dumbbell Lateral Raises for Shoulders

Exercise 4: Barbell Shoulder Press

Exercise 5: Rope Pushdown

Pull

Exercise 1: Cable Lat Pulldown

Exercise 2: Dumbbell Row

Exercise 3: Barbell Bicep Curls

Exercise 4: Cable Shrugs

Exercise 5: Reverse Wrist Curls

Legs

Exercise 1: Dumbbell Romanian Deadlifts

Exercise 2: Machine Seated Leg Extension

Exercise 3: Barbell Squats

Exercise 4: Machine Seated Leg Curls

Exercise 5: Seated Calf Raises

What to eat?

Stay away from DIETS.

This includes every single diet which promises you the results of your dreams in a short period of time. The concept of a diet is the restriction of the amount of food that you eat through various methods. Such as limiting the time in which you are allowed to eat, restricting, or eliminating certain foods, reducing the amount of your food, or starving yourself.

The answer to "What to eat?" is very simple. Try your best to eat as healthy as possible and eat according to your goal.

To lose weight, eat less than what your body needs to maintain its current weight.

To build muscle or gain strength, eat a bit more than what your body needs to maintain its current weight.

To find out how much you should eat you can go online and firstly calculate your BMI. This would be a great starting point as it will show you if you are overweight, underweight or if you have a healthy weight. Majority of people start going to the gym for health reason and want to address those as quick as possible. Unfortunately, there is no quick fix, my recommendation for people which are overweight, underweight is that they should try to align their goals with being as healthy as possible.

After you had a look at your BMI, you should look online for a BMR calculator. Your BMR (Basal Metabolic Rate) is the amount of calories which your body needs to consume to maintain your current weight. As a beginner you will need to track your calories, there are several calorie journals which you can install on your phone and check how much you have consumed.

To lose weight, you should eat between 100 and 500 calories less than your BMR.

To build muscle or gain strength, you should eat between 100 and 500 calories more than your BMR.

The wrong way to start your process is to either eat 500 calories more/ less (depending on your goal) from the beginning of your fitness journey.

The right way to start your fitness journey is by starting at 100 calories more/less (depending on your goal) and making small adjustments over time.

In regards with what food, you should eat I believe that everyone should try to have a variety of foods in their lifestyle and that everyone is different. Therefore, some foods which can be generally considerate healthy might not be as healthy for you. One thing which you should do across your lifestyle is trying to reduce more of the foods which have a negative impact on your body and eat more of the foods which have a positive impact on your body. Most of the time it can be near impossible to detect which foods have a negative impact on our body unless we have a sever allergy or intolerance to a certain food. Majority of people can have small intolerances and allergies which they can live with.

I encourage you to experiment and find out though elimination if there are any foods that affect your current lifestyle.

Test Yourself By Elimination

Firstly, you will need a journal to record how you feel, you can print out this page or just copy the following questions into your journal.

Rate yourself on a scale from one though five, with one being the lowest and five being the highest.

How tired do you feel this morning after waking up?

Extremely Tired   Well Rested

1   2   3   4   5

How hungry did you feel throughout your day?

Extremely Hungry   Not Hungry

1   2   3   4   5

How social did you feel throughout your day?

Extremely Anxious   Very Social

1   2   3   4   5

How would you rate your skin and hair?

Not looking healthy   Quite healthy

1   2   3   4   5

How would you rate your level of
motivation?

Not motivated at all   Extremely motivated

1   2   3   4   5

Secondly, this process will last five weeks, and you will have to complete the above questions every single day.

In the first week you should eat normally and complete those questions. At the end of the week, you should have a look and see how you scored.

Second week you will have to remove sugar from your lifestyle. I know it can be difficult, but processed sugar is found in almost everything today and it has a big impact on your health. Try your best to cut it out from your life for this first week, and record how you are feeling without it. At the end of the week cheek how your body has responded without sugar. Majority of people find that the beginning of the week is quite horrible and that they have extreme cravings, but by the end of the week feel that fruits and veggies change their taste, and they have more energy. A quick trick for those cravings is to use low calories sweeteners, full sugar drinks with no sugar drinks and to replace sweet snacks with sweet fruits.

During the third week it is your choice to add sugar back to your lifestyle or to not consume sugar at all. What you will need to avoid during this week are products which contain milk/lactose. This includes milk, yogurt, cheese, chocolate, anything that contains milk. About half of the entire globe population, it is considerate to be lactose intolerant. By removing milk and effectively lactose for a week you can find out if your body is negatively affected by lactose. If you find yourself missing milk in your coffee, yogurt or cheese have a look for plant-based alternatives such as soya.

Starting your week four, you are in control on how much sugar and milk-based products you consume. My advice is that you should compare your weeks and eat according to how you feel. If you feel better without sugar and/or milk-based products, you should keep them to zero at the moment or maybe in small quantities. For this week you want to avoid to the best of your ability products which contain gluten. Not everyone responds well to gluten, by taking the gluten out of your diet for this week you will get a good idea on how your body responds to without gluten. Continue to record how you feel and get ready for the last week.

Starting week five, which is the last week you should have a good idea on how your body responds without sugar, lactose, and gluten. You are in full control to decide how much of those products you want to eat. My recommendation is that you continue to eat for your goal and try to avoid foods that make you feel bad. This week you are trying to restrict processed food and fast food to see how your body responds in their absence. Processed foods are any product already manufactured that contains several ingredients which preserve their shelve life. You might consider this week to be the hardest week, my recommendation to you is to take this as a game or the opportunity to learn how to cook. You can plan your week ahead and try to make it interesting and exciting. At the end of this week, you will have a god idea how your body responds to processed and fast foods. Together with your experience with excluding sugar, lactose, and gluten you can make informed decision on how some foods affect your health. Remember this is not a diet, the rational or idea behind this process is not to make you lose or gain weight or gain. The rational of this process is to make you aware of your current lifestyle and find out how sugar, lactose, gluten, processed and fast foods affect you.

Design your own Plan

Now it's time you design your own plan, complete, and use the layout underneath, you can print out or copy this in a notebook. Try to be as creative as you want. Set up targets for yourself and create a visual board to inspire and motivate yourself. In the "Choose your goal" section we have explored three different goals, building muscle, becoming more athletic or becoming more powerful. Choose one and stick with it for a good period of time, I recommend one year. In section "Choose your training" decide how many days you can allocate to your goal then have a look at some beginners' routines which we have explored and choose one that fits your schedule.

In the following section "eat for your goal" you need to calculate your BMR and eat accordingly to your goal. Quick reminders start with a deficit or surplus (eat less or more) with about 100 calories and adjust things over time.

Choose your Goal

Choose your Training

Eat for your Goal